This booklet is furnished for your reading pleasure in hopes of making the next nine months a memorable and happy experience.

COMPLIMENTS OF

Your Physician

AND

Reid-Provident Laboratories, Inc.

ATLANTA, GEORGIA

Important Information:

Physician's Name _____

Office Phone Number _____

Nurse's Name _____

Receptionist's Name _____

Hospital Name _____

Drug Store Name _____

Phone Number _____

Personal Notes

_____
_____
_____
_____
_____
_____
_____
_____
_____
_____
_____
_____
_____
_____
_____
_____
_____

A Pregnancy Primer

by

Robert C. Patterson, Jr., M.D.

About the author . . .

Dr. Patterson was graduated from Vanderbilt University Medical School. He is a Founding Fellow of the American College of Obstetricians and Gynecologists. He is an Assistant Clinical Professor of Obstetrics and Gynecology at the Vanderbilt University Medical School.

Copyright © 1973 by
Aurora Publishers, Incorporated
Nashville, Tennessee 37203
Library of Congress Catalog Card Number 72-85160
Standard Book Number 87695-160-4
Manufactured in United States of America

Contents:

Preface   page
1. So you think you are pregnant? 1
2. First visit to the doctor or . . . the
   cold stethoscope 3
3. Subsequent visits to the doctor 8
4. Danger signals of the first three months 11
5. The five most asked questions 13
6. Dispositional changes 17
7. Discomforts of pregnancy 19
8. Diet! 22
9. Complications of pregnancy 26
10. "Alarming accidents" during pregnancy 30
11. Phone calls 32
12. Labor 34
13. Sedation during labor 37
14. Natural childbirth 41
15. Induction of labor 44
16. Delivery 45
17. The RH factor and Rubella vaccination 48
18. The hospital 50
19. The expectant grandmother 52
20. Postpartum hospital course 55
21. Going home 58
22. Old wives' tales and some random facts 64
23. Miscellaneous tips 67
    Shopping list for the baby 69
24. Birth control 70

Preface

Books and pamphlets for the expectant mother are frequently complicated, consisting as they so often do of diagrams with vague explanations. This book offers a practical guide and omits difficult medical terminology which may be misinterpreted.

Your doctor's basic obstretrical textbook is over a thousand pages long, and this barely scratches the surface of the subject. He has had to study many, many volumes and must keep abreast of current trends. His years of training included thousands of hours of discussion with qualified doctors. His practice adds up to years of time-consuming work and study.

How, then, can one small book based upon the scientific approach to pregnancy do much more than leave you uninformed? It can be practical and help you to avoid some of the complications of pregnancy and labor. It can serve as a guide to special questions that you should ask your doctor. It can also prevent needless worry and make you a better patient.

Every pregnancy is different, just as every baby is different. If you understand certain basic facts about your condition, you will feel happier and more secure. Never forget that you are a very definite part of God's greatest work. You are creating and producing life.

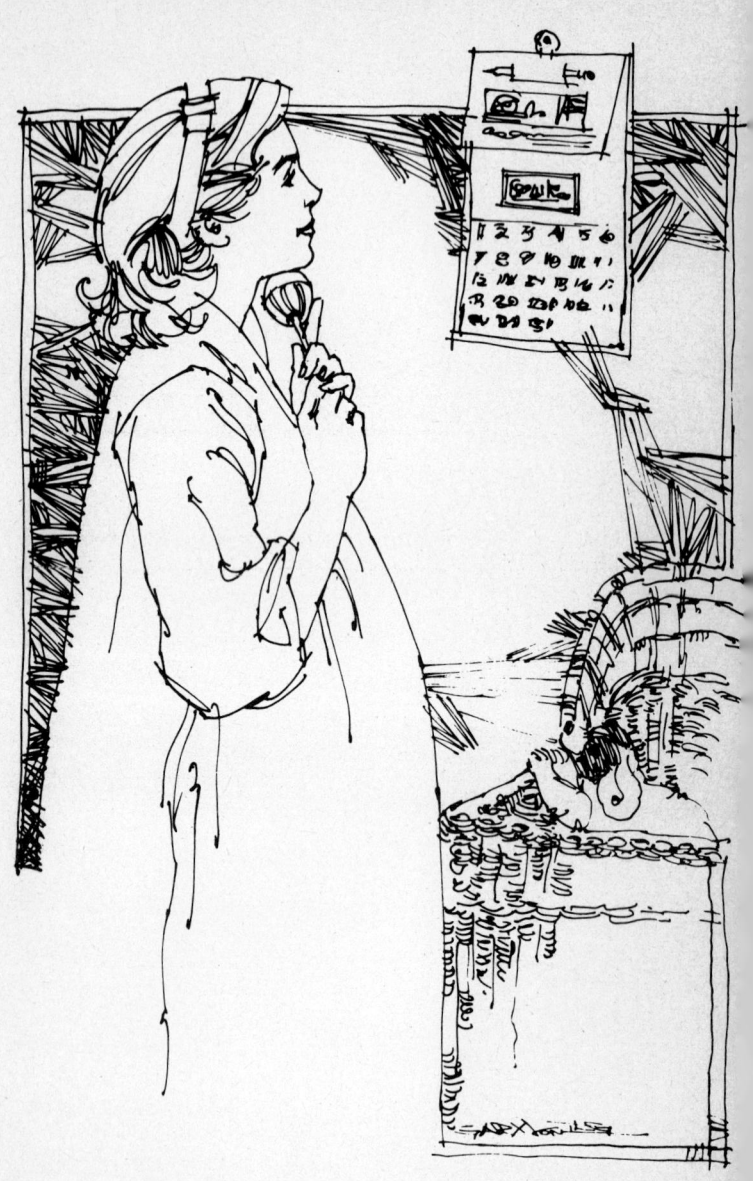

Chapter 1

So you think you are pregnant?

So you think you are pregnant? You dash for the calendar and look for the check-marks denoting your last menstrual period. It is not there. It seldom is. Memory recalls that the last time you menstruated, Aunt Minnie was visiting or you had the bridge club over for lunch. You may think you are as regular as clockwork, but this is not strictly true. An actual graphing of the date over a year's period may show a wide variation in the menstrual cycle. A normal female may vary as much as twenty-five to thirty-five days or, on the other hand, she may show only slight deviation. As you probably know, menstruation is the time when the lining of the womb (uterus) is shed because conception did not take place. Shakespeare called this "the weeping of a disappointed womb."

There are standard guidelines to use in determining whether or not you are pregnant. Though individually these symptoms do not necessarily mean you are pregnant, if they are all present the diagnosis is likely to be positive. In the first two months of pregnancy, the breasts are apt to become tender and slightly enlarged. Frequency of urination is often experienced. You are apt to feel tired and sleepy much of the time, and pure lethargy may set in. It is possible that you may become a bit irritable for no particular reason except that you cannot help it. Some feel a little queasy or unsettled in the stomach, especially in the morning. Cooking breakfast may increase this feeling.

You may sum up the pregnancy possibilities in this ten point way:

		points
1.	Missed a period (any special reason?)	1 point
2.	Breasts sore	1 point
3.	Feel a bit queasy	1 point
4.	Often tired and sleepy	2 points
5.	Frequency of urination	1 point
6.	Cooking in the a.m. increases queasiness	1 point
7.	Irritability for no special reason	1 point
8.	Missed two periods	2 points
	Total	10 points

Total of ten points . . . . you're probably pregnant!

Chapter 2

First visit to the doctor or . . . the cold stethoscope

On your first medical visit a nurse or a doctor will start a chart of your case which will record your age, address, religion et cetera, and also a complete past history of previous pregnancies, menstrual cycle, operations, and illnesses. A family history of you and your husband is often noted. On subsequent visits your weight gain will be recorded, along with other pertinent information concerning the advancement of your pregnancy.

Obstetricians know that every girl is anxious about the first visit to the office. There is absolutely no need for this because anxiety and tension are mental attitudes that can be avoided. The doctor, assisted by a nurse, will give a complete physical examination. In the professional care of a gentle and understanding doctor, there is no reason for embarrassment or discomfort. The examination is necessary for a positive diagnosis of pregnancy, as well as for detecting any abnormal physical condition. Although the gown that the doctor's office supplies for this examination is not a thing of beauty, it prevents undue exposure of the body. This check-up will include heart, lungs, breasts, and the pelvic area. Routine lab work will be processed on a blood sample and urine speciman. Your doctor will discuss the results of these tests on the next visit.

Now how can you make the first examination easy on yourself? You can rationalize over and over that millions of women have been through this and that your doctor probably examines forty patients daily. These thoughts seldom help. After you have put on the gown, looked at the most uncomfortable table you will ever see, you are helped onto the examination table by the nurse, who often gives you pleasant but not soothing words about, "It will be over in just a minute" or "It's a wonderful day outside". The doctor comes in, checks your heart, your lungs, and external areas. A light will be turned on the perineal area (vagina). Your hands will grasp the side of the table. You are very tense and wish that you were at home. This is wrong. Very wrong.

What you should do is simple and easy. Lie down and place your arms at full length by your sides. Have the palms turned up and keep the fingers extended (don't make a fist or hold on to the table). Begin taking deep, regular breaths, and think over and over that your stomach muscles are very relaxed. If you follow this simple routine, there will be **no pain.** Before you realize it, the examination is over. A tense, tightly wound-up patient is difficult to examine. The physician often cannot tell anything owing to the rigidity of the patient's abdominal muscles. Practice this suggested relaxation at home on your bed before going to the office. Again, palms up, deep breaths, and you will say, as I have heard thousands of times, "Is that all there is to it?" Friends can really needle you about this first examination. Why one woman desires to spook another is something that doctors have never understood.

You may not have a positive diagnosis of pregnancy on the first physical findings. Girls have different-sized uteri just as they have different-sized hands and feet. The early size of the womb is not always a positive sign. If in doubt, most physicians have an available test for the urine specimen that can be done in a few minutes. This is fairly accurate.

If you are diagnosed as pregnant, you will be given an Expected Date of Confinement (E.D.C.) on the first visit. This is 280 days from the date of the beginning of your last menstrual period, or substract three calendar months and add seven days to this date and you get the same E.D.C. This is an estimated date of birth. As pregnancy progresses, your doctor may offer further information to correct the expected date.

During the course of this first visit, you will often be given a diet list. You will be warned against greasy foods, including some things you probably enjoy such as barbecue, french fries, fried chicken, chili, and bacon. **These foods cause nausea the next day or earlier.** Just as an excessive drinker suffers from a hangover the next day, so will the pregnant person experience ill effects from greasy foods. The drinker doesn't blame his hangover on getting out of bed, but the pregnant woman who has indulged in greasy foods blames pregnancy for her morning sickness. What she has eaten the day before is the cause.

Here are some other steps to combat or prevent nausea:
1. **Don't allow your stomach to become empty.**
2. **Nibble dry toast and crackers.**
3. **Sip soft drinks.**
4. **Ice chips will help.**
5. **Drugs are available that may prove helpful, but there is no drug that will allow you to eat greasy foods without feeling ill afterwards.**

Nausea generally does not last past the third month, but the greasy foods can cause heartburn and other side effects discussed in the chapter on **DIET**. If you follow your doctor's orders, you may never experience any of these symptoms.

When your first visit is over, it is advisable to get the following items from your drugstore:

1. **Prenatal Vitamins:**
   Your doctor will prescribe vitamins which should be taken until the baby is six weeks old.

2. **Paregoric:**
   Some doctors give you a prescription for paregoric. Take a teaspoonful in water for cramping, pain, or diarrhea.

3. **Milk of Magnesia Tablets, Maalox, Gelusil:**
   These are for indigestion or heartburn. DO NOT TAKE THE FREQUENTLY ADVERTISED FIZZY SODA DRINKS FOR THIS: The sodium bicarbonate content will cause your ankles to swell.

4. **Laxatives:**
   Almost all laxatives are effective. Constipation can't be cured in the pregnant person. A normal bowel action is important.

When you get home, remember what your doctor has told you. Do not listen to your mother, grandmother, or best friend. They have had either the 'hardest" or the "easiest" pregnancy on record because time seems to either enhance or dim their memories. There are more superstitions and old-wives tales connected with pregnancy than with any other physical condition. **ASK YOUR DOCTOR.**

LISTEN ONLY TO YOUR DOCTOR. He has spent years in scientific study and observation. He has seen hundreds of patients. You are unique and very special to him, but the patterns of pregnancy have been well defined for years. He is interested in all your symptoms, but is very apt to have heard them many times before. He has answers for **all** your questions and anxieties about your pregnancy.

On the next visit, your doctor will appreciate your bringing a written list of any questions that you and your husband may have. It is often difficult to remember everything you wanted to ask when you are in the doctor's office. Help yourself and your doctor by making out this list before you come to the office. Strangely enough, much time is consumed by the patient looking off into space and trying to recall some questions she was going to ask. She remembers these questions when she is half way home.

THE FIRST VISIT TO THE DOCTOR

	Points
1. Relax during the examination by deep breathing. (See, it wasn't bad at all.)	4
2. Listen to your doctor.	4
3. Purchase prescribed medicine.	1
4. Begin to follow diet orders.	3
5. If you listen to friends and relatives.	—4 (minus)
6. Begin list of questions for next visit.	2
	10 points

You have a good start!

Chapter 3

Subsequent visits to the doctor . . .

The second visit to your doctor is usually a month after your first visit. The monthly visits will continue until you are thirty weeks pregnant (thirty weeks from the start of your last menstrual period). From thirty weeks until the E.D.C. they will be more often and when near term, they may be weekly.

Each visit will entail your bringing a urine specimen collected that morning. Most doctors receive small containers for this purpose from a pharmaceutical house, and they will furnish them for you. Collecting the specimen is quite easy with a plastic funnel purchased from a dime store. When the nurse calls you into the examining area, give her the specimen.

The nurse will weigh you, take your blood pressure, and probably add some bits of advice. She will then take you to one of the examining rooms. The doctor will check your stomach to see how high the uterus is in the abdomen and if it is at the navel, he will listen for the baby's heart beat (the foetal heart tone or F.H.T.) This is first heard through the doctor's head stethoscope when you are halfway through your pregnancy. This is usually about the twentieth week, but there is some variation in each patient. Several electronic devices are available which detect the baby's heartbeat much earlier. After the examination, the doctor will give you additional instructions. **Now is the time for your list of questions.** Again, don't have the long, long pause with the murmuring of, "There was something I had to ask you, but I've forgotten."

As you approach term, the doctor will be able, by checking your abdomen, to determine the position of the baby **at that moment.** The baby moves over and around, changing positions until he is firmly engaged in the pelvis. The doctor will tell you when this condition exists.

Friends often inform you that you are carrying your baby low. Don't argue with them. Eighty-five percent of babies do not "drop" (become engaged in the pelvis) until labor begins. The fifteen percent of women whose babies drop earlier have no advantage over their sisters who are in the majority. There is no set number of days from the time the baby drops (lightening is the technical term) until you go into labor. The guess would extend from ten days to three weeks, but even this varies. The doctor cannot tell you the exact date of birth. He guesses.

As the date of confinement approaches, the doctor will explain in detail when to 'phone him concerning your going to the hospital. He will give you a step-by-step description of what happens to you from the time you enter the hospital until your baby is born.

When the baby is well-engaged, the doctor may do a very gentle pelvic examination to determine the condition of the cervix (the opening of the womb). This may give him additional information as to the delivery date and the comparative size of your pelvic bones and the baby's presenting part. The pelvic examination may cause a little spotting of blood, but don't be alarmed.

If this is your first baby, quite a few doctors want you to bring your husband to the office. Make an appointment sometime during the eighth or ninth month for this. Tell the receptionist in advance when your husband will be coming with you so that she can allocate extra time for the visit. After the doctor has examined you, he can talk to both of you in his office.

The visit will be made as easy as possible on your husband. The most self-possessed of husbands are embarrassed when sitting in a room filled with pregnant women. They don't want to stare absent-mindedly at any of the other patients, and they don't know what to do with their eyes, their hands, or their laughter at something you said.

Chapter 4

Danger signals of the first three months . . .

Vaginal spotting or bleeding—with or without cramping. Twenty women out of every hundred threaten to lose their babies in early pregnancy. This is first recognized by vaginal spotting or bleeding. It is often accompanied by pain similar to menstrual cramps or the feeling just before a period. AT THE FIRST SIGN OF THIS, GO TO BED. Most patients panic. The response of friends and relatives often adds to the tension of the situation. Complete bed rest is necessary during the period of spotting or bleeding, and for forty-eight hours after it stops.

Many patients call their doctor and want something done. An immediate examination would please patients because they feel the doctor is doing all he can, but a pelvic examination during the **first several hours** of bleeding may actually help to bring on the threatened miscarriage. Your doctor may wish to do such an examination several days later.

For Abdominal Cramping: Take a teaspoonful of paregoric in a glass of water, and repeat every hour or so if needed.

11

You cannot overdo this with the prescription your doctor has given you. Absolute bed rest until your doctor says otherwise.

Presence of mind and paregoric save many babies. It is a fact that blood is red and, if passed at night, doubly stimulates fear and anxiety. Patients often call to say that they are hemorrhaging. They are rushed to the hospital because of exaggerating the condition. If you pass a blood clot the size of an orange, save it and call your doctor.

An old wives tale says that bleeding is the way in which Mother Nature throws off an imperfect production of conception. This is often salve for the patient's feelings who has lost her baby. After the initial bleeding, you may go to your doctor's office for weekly medications to help you to carry the baby. Would any doctor give medication to save a deformed baby? Of course not.

Vaginal Bleeding:

1. Go to bed.
2. Do not panic.
3. Notify your doctor at his office.
4. Remain in bed until your doctor tells you to get up.
5. If the orange-sized clot is passed, **save it** and call your doctor at once.

If a miscarriage is experienced once, it does not mean that all of your pregnancies will end in this manner. Each pregnancy is different, and your doctor will do several uncomplicated tests to check whether or not certain physical conditions added to the cause.

Chapter 5

The five most asked questions

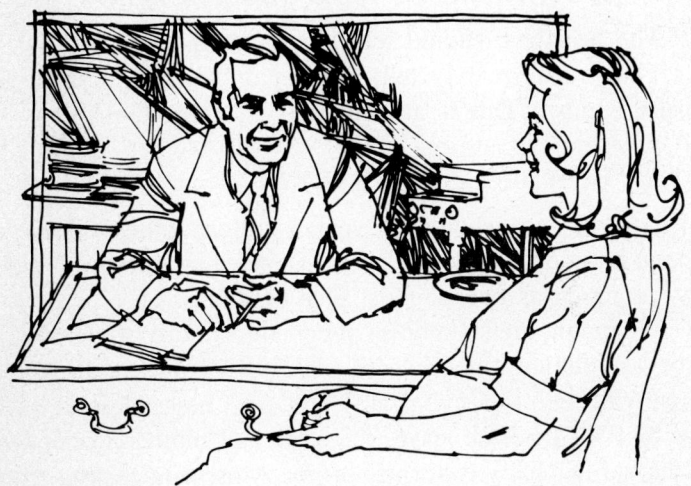

1. "WHEN IS MY BABY DUE?"

The obstetrician can make a guess, and I mean a guess, as you approach term. He cannot tell you the exact date until you start into labor. The Expected Date of Confinement (E.D.C.) is explained in Chapter 2. It takes a different amount of time to "make" babies, just as ovulation (fertile period) varies in each woman. Even if you know the exact time of conception, the doctor will only be able to guess at the time of birth. Please don't ask the question over and over on each visit. The doctor knows you are very, very anxious to have your baby. He knows it has been a long nine months. He knows that friends are calling you daily and asking, "Haven't you gone yet?" He knows that friends are telling you about women who never went into labor and "the doctor had to bring the baby on". The doctor probably induced labor because the patient was exhausted, mentally and physically, by the pressure of the many calls. See Chapter 15 on Induction of Labor.

2. "IS IT GOING TO BE A GIRL OR A BOY?

The heartbeat should tell you something."
The heartbeat only tells the doctor whether or not the baby is alive. This is all that is really important.

3. "HOW BIG IS MY BABY?"

Doctors can usually tell you if you are going to have a large baby or a very small one. Doctor can guess and miss by as much as two pounds, plus or minus.

When you are six months pregnant or more (if you aren't the fat patient), helpful friends and relatives will worry you with such statements as, "You can't be as close to term as that!" This often leaves the expectant mother wondering whether her baby is normal or not. Most women who have had babies think they are an expert on all affairs dealing with pregancy, labor, and related subjects. The fact that you have had teeth pulled does not make you a dentist; the fact that you have had a baby does not make you an authority on labor or pregnancy. Each case is different. Friends always exaggerate their own experiences. To prove my point, try telling them something about your case **before** the baby is born, and they will interrupt to tell you about **their case.**

4. "WHEN WILL I FEEL MY BABY MOVE?"
(Or the Gymnastic Foetus)

You usually feel the baby kick at twenty weeks from the start of the last menstrual period. The time may vary by as much as three weeks, plus or minus; each pregnancy is different.

You may think you feel this first sign of life before you actually do. The confusion is caused by the growth of the uterus. Originally a pelvic organ, it has now expanded into the abdominal cavity and is about the size of a large grapefruit. As the foetus grows into the abdominal area, the small intestines are pushed not only up, but also outward toward the wall of the stomach muscles. The intestines have constant waves of peristalisis to move the food toward the lower bowel. At times a small loop of intestines may get so near the abdominal wall that one feels a flutter, which may be confused with the first kicking of the foetus (quickening).

As soon as your doctor hears the foetal heart tone (F.H.T.), he will tell you. This is life. It is exciting. A short time later, you may allow your husband to place his hand on your abdomen and "feel him kick". (Incidentally, the husband's sperm determines the sex of the baby. It is never "her" before birth for some strange reason.)

You may feel pulsations through the abdomen in the later stages of pregnancy. This is not the baby's heartbeat. It is the uterus pressing on the larger blood vessels that are under it. It is normal. This pulsation is the same as one's heartbeat or pulse.

Some doctors have an instrument that allows the patient to hear the baby's heartbeat as well as the blood going through the placenta (afterbirth). When the small bell of the instrument is placed against your abdomen, the sound of the foetus' heartbeat is projected loud and clear into the examining room. Patients can often hear the heartbeat when they are only twelve-weeks pregnant. Obese patients with thick abdominal walls will hear this sign of life at a later date. The instrument also gives a fairly accurate diagnosis of twins.

5. "IS MY BABY ALL RIGHT?"

One of the most important questions that patients think but do not ask directly is whether or not the baby is all right. Every (and I repeat every) mother worries about this. This worry is usually not even voiced to the husband. The expectant mother gets premonitions that her baby is going to be abnormal. This varies from a horrible deformity to having a small toe turned in. The suppressed worry demonstrates itself by sly questions to the doctor: "Is my baby growing normally?" "Am I as large as I should be?" "Is my baby in the correct position?"

This unnecessary worry is often stimulated by friends ("You couldn't be as far as that! You aren't big enough!") Unintentionally they seem to be implying that something is wrong with your unborn child. They don't think of the doubt they have planted in your already anxious mind.

If your doctor thinks you are going to have a malformed child, it is because there are some signs that give him a suspicion of this fact. HE WILL DISCUSS THEM WITH YOU. He doesn't hide anything from you. I suggest that you come forward with a frank question. Ask him if your baby is showing any signs of abnormal prenatal development. New techniques (still in the early stages of development) may eventually result in prenatal detection of chromosome abnormalities and inborn errors of metabolism which produce the very rare abnormal child. The technical term for these studies is amniocentesis. The analysis of amniotic fluid (the water in which the foetus floats) may reveal a malformed infant. I should stress that this study is very theoretical and has many years to go before malformity is discovered prior to birth, but I truthfully tell patients that they are fifty times more likely to be struck by a car while crossing a street than to have a deformed child.

Chapter 6

Dispositional changes

I would estimate that half the pregnant girls do not wish to "be with child". Even in this time of scientific birth control, many pregnancies are unplanned. Don't have a guilt feeling, and don't pretend to others. Just say, "I'm expecting" and don't comment. This rejection of the baby happens to many women and usually diminishes when they feel the baby move. It is a transient attitude which is stimulated by such things as changes in hormones, financial troubles, planned trips or other children.

There is a tremendous feeling of lethargy in early pregnancy. This will remain in varying degrees throughout the 280 days. You may feel tired for a week, then you may experience a sudden burst of energy! This latter is called the nesting instinct. You frequently return to the sleepy stage again.

Irritability is often experienced until the birth of the baby. This varies in intensity and seems to increase as one nears term. You are apt to get unduly disturbed with everyone. Service personnel such as gas station attendants, salesgirls in the store, and the supermarket checkout man are frequent targets. And then there is your husband. In the eyes of all sympathizing relatives, he is the cause of it all. Added stimulation from them may cause you to nag him unjustly.

The expectant father often comes home from the office after a rather trying day and asks, "How do you feel?" Unfortunately, you can become unglued at this question. Rarely will he just get the silent treatment. The well-intentioned remark often brings a tearful prelude to nagging and complaining. His sincere "How do you feel?" is taken as speaking out of turn, being sarcastic, or you name it, it's there.

Husbands must understand that this is a normal course of events. It is believed that the complete change in the hormones during pregnancy is the underlying cause. I suggest that all fathers take everything that is verbally dished out for six days and twenty-three hours a week. For the remaining hour he may blast back verbally, and then retreat into his shell again. Neither partner should remember these spats. They do not hurt the baby, who is probably smiling at the whole mess he has caused. After the birth of your baby, your hormones will be back to normal gear, and so will your disposition. Motherhood brings patience and love in increasing amounts. Fathers must hustle to grow in maturity too.

The Husband

The father-to-be is short-tempered and rather tense and tries to hide this from you. He worries all day about **you** and **his** baby. He thinks horrible thoughts about an emergency in which he has to deliver the baby at home. His jovial friends at the office are no help. When their wives were pregnant, they received a bit of needling from him. He is getting it back, but doesn't understand because **his** wife and **his** child are involved. He can't tell anyone (and I mean anyone) that he is worrying about two of his dearest possessions—his wife and his baby-to-be. So, when he comes home, he too is uptight. The word-battle often starts. Please understand that he is disturbed. His nonchalance is a cloak to hide his worries about you. Don't think that it is indifference; it isn't. He just doesn't want to tell you he is upset, for he thinks that this would be just another burden for you.

Chapter 7

Discomforts of pregnancy

Pressure Pains:

You will experience pressure pains as the baby grows larger. These manifest themselves by pain in the groin, across the bladder "low down", hip pain, numbness down one leg, or backache from walking erectly. The baby is pressing down and out. You do not want to walk bent over, so you unconsciously arch your back. This causes pain across the lower back, as well as between the shoulder blades. It hurts, but is not dangerous.

Every pregnant woman experiences these, and much time is consumed in explaining them to the patient when the doctor should be giving more important instructions. Realize that you are continuing the miraculous process of creation. It is a great gift. Two microscopic cells develop in the uterus to become a human. Let's see NASA in Texas match that. They can't.

Prevention: The force of gravity is naturally down. If you stand or sit, the baby is pressing downward. To prevent this or at least stall off its occurrence, understand that the only way you can rest is by reclining. A pillow under the small of your back with your feet on the armrest of a sofa is excellent.

Every doctor hears about pressure pains in great detail, and the pregnant one ends up by saying, "I didn't do anything yesterday." Questioning reveals such activities as sitting and talking with friends, a shopping trip, a too-long drive, or the like. Don't forget that these pains are not dangerous but are bothersome and preventable. Follow the routine of RECLINING rest for thirty minutes out of every two hours, or some comparable schedule.

Sex Drives:

Soon after you conceive, you realize that you no longer desire intercourse. The desire becomes less and less as pregnancy advances. This is normal; it is due to the hormonal change, plus your subconscience fear that the male organ is near your baby. Watching television or playing cards becomes the pastime. Your husband probably puts up a pretty good show of "suffering". Tell him to take a cold bath and forget it. Intercourse causes some pain from the fifth month on due to the engorgment of the blood vessels of the vagina, which is preparing for childbirth.

Research has shown that if the female reaches a climax, there is a temporary lack of oxygen going to the foetus. This apparently does not harm the baby, but it is suggested that intercourse be restricted to only once a week and stopped after the thirtieth week of pregnancy. Obviously, if any bleeding is experienced, there should be no intercourse until instructed otherwise by your doctor.

Cystitis:

Cystitis is often called a bladder or kidney infection by your friends. The symptoms are FREQUENCY, URGENCY (when you have to go, you have to go), and BURNING of urination.

Treatment: In the early stages of this disorder, drink copious amounts of water. This often takes care of the uncomfortable condition. No female drinks an adequate supply of water. Coffee, tea, and cokes, YES: but water, NO. Mention your symptoms to your doctor and he may wish to give you an antibiotic. In late pregnancy the spasms and pain of the bladder from this condition often makes you think you are in labor. If this is your second baby or more, a twenty-four hour stay in the hospital may be necessary in order to differentiate between cystitis and labor.

IRRITATING VAGINAL DISCHARGE:

Some vaginal discharge (other than blood) is often seen in pregnancy. This can either be mild or very irritating. Prevention is easier than treatment. Cotton panties worn throughout the nine months will be helpful. Synthetic fibers increase the temperature of the vagina, often causing an excessive growth of the vaginal contaminates. Douche powders, sprays, and lack of ventilation partially cause and aggravate this condition.

Mention this discharge to your doctor on your next visit. He may prescribe something for this uncomfortable condition. If the irritation occurs suddenly at night, use a vinegar-and-water wash. A mixture of two tablespoonsful of vinegar to a quart of water poured over the outside of the vagina will prove soothing.

HEMORRHOIDS:

Hemorrhoids are dilated veins around the rectum. The causes are twofold:
1. Constipation
2. The normal pressure of the unborn baby downward against the blood return to the upper body.

Treatment: Any of the topical ointments are good for temporary relief. Hot tub baths (sitz baths) several times a day are better. If one of the hemorrhoids turn **black,** call your doctor. He will make an incision and express a small blood clot the size of a pea. The pain of these black hemorrhoids can be bad, and you welcome anything that is done for them; however, they are not dangerous.

Prevention: (1) A normal bowel action. (2) Elevate your feet several times a day for ten to fifteen minutes. Early treatment with the sitz baths and ointments will prevent black blood clots (thrombotic hemorrhoids).

Chapter 8

DIET!

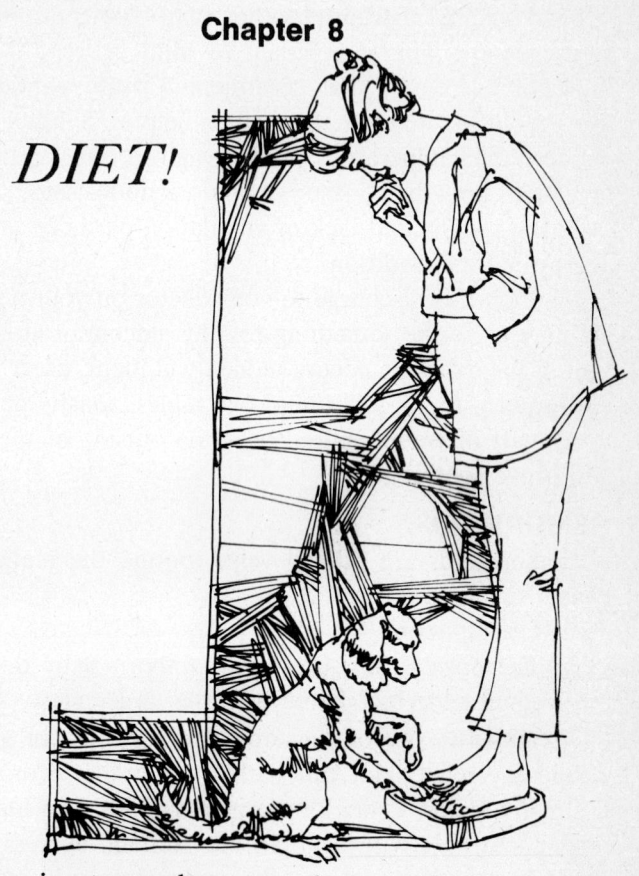

Hunger is a tremendous urge of pregnancy. Your doctor will give you the correct diet and help you watch your weight. For the average patient, eighteen pounds is enough to gain. Never forget that your appetite can get you and your baby into trouble.

Friends and relatives will tempt you with goodies. You will be offered snacks every time you see the girl friends.

You will be told that you must eat for two. There will be special occasions that will tempt you (Christmas, Thanksgiving, birthdays, wedding parties, picnics, etc.) These are excuses to overeat, but not the cause. Friends and relatives who encourage you to break your diet "just this one time" are (1) not present when delivery is taking place, (2) have no responsibility for the outcome of your case, and (3) do not realize the complications of excess weight gain.

Follow the diet given below. It allows you to eat all you want within reason. No doctor wants to starve you, but he will insist that you adhere to a HIGH PROTEIN, low fat, low carbohydrate diet.

The diet list below is suggested instead of counting calories for the following reasons:

1. It is tedious to list every bite one takes. The measuring of **exact** amounts of food and certain drinks is necessary for an accurate calorie count.

2. From the fourth month of pregnancy to term, you have very little will power. If you take a small piece of apple pie, you will often eat the whole pie.

3. A "do and don't" diet is easily remembered and cuts down on temptation and hunger.

DIET LIST

Dairy Products: Buttermilk; fat-free milk; diet ice cream, or sherbet; cottage cheese; yogurt.

Eggs: Cooked anyway except in animal fat.

Meats: Lean beef (NO LIVER or other animal organs); chicken (not fried in animal fat) with the skin removed after cooking. This omits most luncheon meats, hot dogs, bologna, spreads, and the like.

Vegetable Products: Most vegetables are good for you, but the manner in which they are cooked can do you harm. If you cook string beans (avoid lima and pinto beans) with a portion of bacon, it is the same as eating that portion of bacon. Avoid starchy vegetables such as corn and potatoes.

Seafoods: Good for you; but again, don't fry in animal fat.

Beverages: Water and unsweetened juices should be taken in copious amounts. Coffee and tea, soft drinks in moderate amounts only. Soups which do not form a covering of grease when cooled are allowed. Watch out for friends bringing you a "nourishing bowl of soup" which they think will calm your nausea and give you strength. It is often like pouring gasoline on a fire.

Fruits: Fruits are excellent in large amounts. Wash the syrup off canned fruits or use the good dietary products available.

A recent article in a popular magazine suggested that the pregnant person be allowed to eat all and everything she desired in order to prevent mental hangups during the nine months. You should recall two things; no article is going to talk with you and your husband if things don't go normally. Too, such an article is merely a crutch for the weak-willed patient. Again, your doctor is responsible and he will give you all the advice you need. This article was only one man's idea, and a psychologist's at that.

COMPLICATIONS CAUSED IN PART OR TOTALLY BY OBESITY DURING PREGNANCY

1. **Toxemia:** Blood pressure is up. Feet are swollen in the evenings. Face and hands are swollen in the mornings. Some albumin is present in the urine specimen. This condition develops in a matter of days. Although office visits are weekly when near term, you can develop toxemia between

visits. Toxemia can result in convulsions and a stillborn baby. This is a **preventable** complication caused by YOU.

2. **Difficult Delivery:** Fat accumulates not only outwardly on your body, but also inwardly. This impinges on the birth canal, causing soft tissue dystocia. The term means that fat reduces the space between the pelvic bones that is needed by the baby during delivery.

3. **Stitches hurt more:** The doctor must cut through an inch or more of fat before the **resisting structures** are met. Obviously, this means more sewing. Moreover, fatty tissue does not heal as quickly as healthy tissue.

4. **Uterine Inertia:** The fat globules invade the wall of the uterus. Although the contractions are as great as in normal labor, their effectiveness is greatly reduced. This causes inertia or the stopping of the needed contractions to move the baby along. In some cases a Caesarean section has to be performed just BECAUSE THE PREGNANT ONE DID NOT CONTROL HER APPETITE.

5. **Appearance:** Excessive weight gained during pregnancy leaves the mother looking pregnant after the baby is born. This does not make too much difference to the doctor, but it does to the husband and girl. A once-shapely young girl has lost her eye-appeal.

Many doctors do not **stress** diet enough. They do not wish to offend you and cause you to change doctors. You must remember that anything your doctor says is for **your** good as well as your baby's. If you saw a two-year-old child walking toward an open fireplace, you would stop him even if he screamed and threw a tantrum. In a similar way, the doctor is trying to keep you from walking as directly and innocently into trouble.

Chapter 9

Complications of pregnancy...

Some Rare, Some More Frequent

The following complications are listed as clearly and simply as possible without too many technical details. It is important for you to know precisely which ones indicate an emergency so that you will know when to 'phone your doctor. Make your diagnosis from the listings below. Your doctor wants to know about these complications.

Miscarriage: (Called a spontaneous abortion in the first few weeks of pregnancy.)

If you pass a blood clot the size of an orange, SAVE THE BLOOD CLOT and 'phone your doctor. There are usually hard abdominal crampings before the clot is expelled. Please don't allow slight bleeding like a menstrual flow panic you into exaggerating the amount passed. This complication does not require an ambulance with sirens to rush you to the hospital or doctor's office. If the large clot you have saved is found to contain tissue, your doctor will perform a D and C procedure to remove the unexpelled products of conception. This requires only overnight hospitalization and you will probably be able to return to normal activity in a few days or a week.

Excessive Bleeding During the Last Two Months of Pregnancy:

If you have definite **flooding** (not spotting or mild vaginal bleeding), call your doctor. He may hospitalize you to determine the location of the afterbirth. If it is in the uterus in front of the baby, a Caesarean section may have to be performed. The first episode of this PAINLESS bleeding is not dangerous. Your doctor may keep you absolutely off your feet to allow the baby to approach term before he operates. The foetus grows better in your uterus than it does in a premature nursery.

Excessive Pain with Tight Abdomen and Bleeding:

Here we stress that this pain is rough. It is not moderate, and it does not come and go. It hits suddenly. The abdomen is hard and remains so. Some textbooks describe this pain as a pain that "knocks" the patient to her knees. This rare condition is accompanied by bleeding and is an emergency. It is termed "abruptio placenta" (the afterbirth is separating from the uterine wall abruptly). If there is not total separation, a live baby can often be saved by an immediate Casearean Section. This is one of the real emergencies of obstetrics, though fortunately very rare, and is easily diagnosed by your doctor.

Premature Labor:

See instructions about full-term labor (Chapter 12). The contractions are the same. Your doctor will hospitalize you. Many patients confuse these pains with the following:

(a) Bladder Spasm: The pains caused by bladder spasm are accompanied by LOW abdominal cramping and frequency of urination. There is a strong urge to urinate, but very little urine is expelled. There is often burning before, after, or during the stream. Treat this by drinking large quantities of water and juices. Take paregoric for pain. Your doctor can also prescribe a helpful drug. This is not an emergency.

(b) Pressure Pains: See Chapter 7.

Rupture of the Bag of Waters:

This is often confused with an involuntary spilling of urine from the bladder. This leakage of water (or **fluid** may be a better word here) is rather common and doesn't mean that the baby is going to be born at once, as friends will so often tell you. No tub baths, intercourse, or douches. Drink fluids in large quantities until your doctor makes the diagnosis in his office the next day (if it happens in the middle of the night). Many patients void involuntarily while asleep because the baby has pressed against the bladder neck. The tone of the bladder and the urge are reduced in pregnancy. Patients are sure that the "waters" have ruptured, and they run to the hospital for an overnight stay. They go home the next day depressed or embarrassed because of this bed-wetting. Don't panic because it is during the night. The light of day plus the above instructions can save you an unnecessary trip to the hospital.

Swelling of the Ankles:

This will occur in most pregnant girls especially during the summer season. Leave salt out of your diet altogether, as your doctor has told you. Mention this swelling to him on the next prenatal visit.

Passing the Mucous Plug, or Blood Show:

Here again girl friends will tell you that labor is really starting. In fact, this can occur a week or so before you start into labor. IGNORE IT AND WAIT FOR THE CONTRACTIONS as described in "Labor" (Chapter 12).

Fainting:

Lie down and get cool. This does not harm the baby. (See explanation in Chapter 10.)

After the Sixth Month, and You Don't Feel the Baby Move:
If you are busy, you may not be conscious of the baby's kicking. Wait twenty-four hours, and "he" will start kicking again. If still worried, go to your doctor's office.

Heartburn and Excessive Gas:
You've been eating greasy foods. Take Maalox, Gelusil, or Milk of Magnesia tablets. Again, DO NOT TAKE ONE OF THE HIGHLY ADVERTISED FIZZY DRINKS. The sodium content of such drinks will cause your ankles to swell.

Leg Cramps:
Tell your doctor about leg cramps on a prenatal visit. An antihistamine taken at bedtime often stops these painful contractions in your calves. (Why this works, I do not know; but it does.)

Chapter 10

"Alarming accidents" during pregnancy...

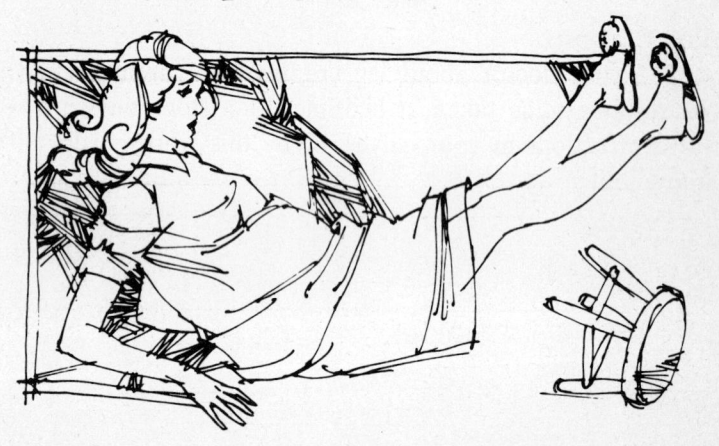

Most pregnant girls experience one or all of the following accidents:

1. **Falling**

Falling may be associated with fainting, but the usual fall does **not** harm the baby. It may sprain the patient's arm or ankle, but God protects the baby by suspending him in a fluid. The baby can take a fall much better than the pregnant mother. Check yourself for sprains and bruises. If fainting is associated with the fall, the patient pushes the panic button: "Call the doctor . . . Call the ambulance . . .

Call my husband home from work!" All of these calls are unnecessary. If you have been feeling the baby move and still feel movement after the fall, you may rest assured that no injury has been done to the foetus.

The bathtub and stairs are the most usual causes of a fall. Take the precaution of using a rubber mat with suction cups for the bathtub. Go up and down stairs cautiously.

2. **Fainting**

Four major causes of fainting are:

Being on your feet for too long a period.

Getting up very suddenly from a reclining or sitting position.

Being in a hot, stuffy place.

Getting overheated.

3. **The Male Elbow in the Tummy During the Night**

Don't panic. Push him back to his side of the bed.

4. **Car Accidents**

If not of a serious nature, car accidents do not harm babies. For some unknown reason, your attorney will not let you sign a release until after the baby is born (attorneys think doctors are "far-out" and vice versa). Seat belts should be worn UNDER THE BABY, NOT ON TOP.

5. **Emotional Shocks**

Shocks do not start labor pains, nor do they "mark the baby". If someone dear to you has a tragedy, call the doctor. He will prescribe a tranquilizer. In case of a death or serious injury in the family, remember your condition. Do not exhaust yourself.

Chapter 11

Phone calls . . .

This chapter could be entitled "How to Receive More Information from Your Doctor" or "How to be a Good Patient". The suggestions below are very important.

YOU SHOULD CALL—not your husband, mother, sister, or friend. The reason for phoning may seem obvious to them, but the doctor usually wants to ask some further questions about your complaint, and the person substituting for you on the phone will not have the answers. Besides, the doctor's instructions should be given directly to the patient. You do not need a well-meaning intermediary.

1. **Phone Calls to the Office**

Always tell the receptionist (a) who you are (b) your complaint (c) your phone number, and (d) your drugstore phone number. If you have an emergency, your doctor will answer immediately. For routine telephone questions, the doctor will usually return the call within thirty minutes after your chart and message are placed on his desk. This short delay should not cause you irritation. How would you have felt if he had interrupted your examination to answer a routine call? Headaches, vomiting, some vaginal spotting of blood, back pain, and the like are not dire emergencies (see previous chapters about these complaints). (It is bad judgement to withhold this information from the doctor's receptionist.) Many doctors receive calls from "friends" of the patient asking if she is due to come to the office. They say, "I am Mrs. Jane Jones's aunt, and I want to tell you what she has been doing." These busybodies are sometimes trying to discover whether or not their friend is pregnant. Often they are "do-gooders" who have no concept of medical ethics.

2. Phone Calls to the Doctor's Home

After many years of practice and many hours of listening to other obstetricians talk, I have found that the most frequent time for home telephone calls is near the evening dinner hour. The cause? The father-to-be has arrived home from work, and his wife tells him all her complaints. He is hungry. He is tired. He demands that she call her doctor. She refuses, so he does the calling. Breaking through the language barrier with an expectant father on the subject of his wife's symptoms is a lost cause. Please make these calls during office hours before your husband comes home; your treatment will be more thorough as the doctor will have your chart on his desk.

For an emergency, or if doubt is in your mind after you have glanced through this primer, call your doctor. When he answers, tell him the following (this is very important):

(a) Your name.
(b) When your baby is due (E.D.C.).
(c) The nature of your complaint.

Speak rather slowly, especially if it is in the middle of the night. Remember, he may be in a deep sleep because of the hours spent at the hospital the previous night. You have been awake and are alert. Your doctor often has several patients with a similar-sounding name. Your speaking slowly gives him the chance to get your name correctly and to get his brain cells in high gear. Telling him the EDC does not mean that he does not know your case, but in the middle of the night he may not recall this quickly. Have your drugstore's telephone number at hand in case he wants to call a prescription. If it is very late, he will probably know of an all-night drugstore.

Chapter 12

Labor . . .

Labor pains are caused by the regular contractions of the muscular part of the uterus, which force the presenting part of the baby against the mouth of the womb. The baby's head is a dilating wedge which is rythemically (with each contraction) pushed against the cervix to dilate it, allowing the baby to pass from the uterus to the birthcanal (vagina). The muscles of the uterus are involuntary muscles which is the reason one cannot strengthen them by exercise either during or before pregnancy.

Contractions start either in the back or in the abdomen and have the following characteristics:
1. They are regular contractions.
2. The pain associated with them is mild at first and builds up with each additional contraction.
3. Walking between or during contractions does not stop the pain (it often does in false labor). In order to feel contractions, place the palms of your hands on your exposed abdomen near the sides of the navel.

When you have established that real labor is in progress you can alleviate the pain by relaxing. This is done by extending your arms by your side, palms up, and taking deep breaths throughout the entire contraction. Practice this on your bed as you approach term. A true labor pain lasts slightly over a minute.

A good rule to follow is:

1. With the first baby call your doctor when you have regular contractions every FIVE minutes for an HOUR.
2. With the second baby plus, call your doctor when the contractions are ten minutes apart, or when you are fairly sure your labor has started.

With first babies there are two basic reasons for going to the hospital too early; (a) false labor, (b) the anxiety of the family when the nine months wait is almost over.

False labor is the tightening of the womb causing some degree of pain, especially across the bladder area. The contractions are irregular. They may come every two minutes, then up to twenty minutes, and again back in two minutes. These contractions, like the real thing, are best felt by placing the palms of your hands (not your fingers) on your abdomen. A spotting of blood is occasionally observed and this rings the panic button in the household. One rule with FIRST babies is to wait until the contractions are REGULAR for at least five minutes for one hour. The timing should be done by the clock, not by guess work.

I may say that I have never had a patient give birth to a first baby before going to the hospital. I have had hundreds of them go several times in false labor. When this occurs the patient goes home after staying in the hospital overnight, or else she is in the hospital for some twenty-odd hours before true labor begins.

The husband is often over-eager to take his wife to the hospital. He is the boss of the family (so he thinks). He can imagine himself delivering his own baby, a duty for which he is totally unprepared. Mother-to-be you have talked to your doctor about when to call him and he has explained much to you. Your husband perhaps has had one conference with the doctor. Be wary of mothers, sisters, and friends too: they often suffer from instant panic. There are two traditional statements that friends will make. The first is that they had a thirty-hour plus labor. (The fact is that they went to the hospital too early). The second is that they were in labor and did not know it. (The fact is that this doesn't happen with first babies)

With second babies plus, call your doctor when you think you are in labor. It may be false labor, bladder spasm, or the like, but he would rather hear from you than have an out-of-hospital birth.

If you **think** that labor is beginning it is very important that you do NOT eat any solid food. You may keep your fluids up. Any anaesthesia given to the patient with food in her stomach is dangerous because food particles may be aspirated into the lungs.

Chapter 13

Sedation during labor . . .

There is no need to experience undue pain during the birth of a baby. Your doctor knows that you have heard exaggerated accounts of childbirth. Let me repeat you will never see a mother who did not have either the hardest or the easiest time in labor and childbirth.

With this in mind, the following basic methods of sedation are presented. It is suggested that you discuss them with your doctor on one of the later prenatal visits.

1. **Medication—oral and injections.**
2. **Regional anaesthesias.**
3. **Natural childbirth (see the following chapter)**
4. **A combination of any of the above.**

Your doctor has the following responsibilities with regard to anaesthesia and analgesia:

1. **To relieve you of undue pain.**
2. **To prescribe drugs that will not harm the baby.**
3. **To prescribe drugs that will not harm you.**

As suggested in Chapter 3, it is an excellent idea to take your husband to the doctor's for a prearranged appointment about four weeks from your "guessed" date of confinement. This is very important with your first baby. After your doctor has given you a tentative plan for relieving your discomfort in labor and delivery, ask the questions you have listed. The usual two questions are "I won't get a spinal, will I?" and "You don't use twilight sleep do you?". The doctor will explain his plan for your case. Of course, unforseen developments may occur between the time you leave the office and the time you go into labor, a few weeks, or even days later. In this eventuality, the regime may vary.

The obstetrician must individualize each case. The plan outlined to you and the expectant father is not inflexible: it is the routine to be followed if your case develops as the doctor expects. He has no crystal ball to predict several of the few minor variables that the patients present. But he will follow the three points mentioned above concerning pain and harm to you and the baby.

If the expectant grandmother is to be at the hospital, it is important to bring her to the office too. She will not write questions down, but will often tell your doctor all about her deliveries. Caution her about this. Remind her that this is **your labor, your delivery** and **your baby.**

As you approach the end of the nine months the cervix is dilated to approximately one half inch in diameter (called two centimeters). To allow the birth of a term baby, the cervix must dilate to ten-plus centimeters (about five fingers breadth) so that the baby can pass from the uterus to the birth canal. The patient cannot control this involuntary muscle (uterus), so even though she is relaxed there will be some pain from the contractions. These can be alleviated in several ways.

MEDICATIONS—ORAL AND INJECTIONS

There are many pain killing drugs available that will not harm you or the baby. Prescribing for the early phase of labor relieve your tension and discomfort. Hypodermic injections are often given when you are some four centimeters dilated (two fingers). The contractions are usually every two to three minutes and last over forty-five seconds. The first injection dulls the pain. When it is wearing off and you are six centimeters dilated (three fingers), you will receive the second shot, which will make you drowsy. All patients think they will say something in this stage of sedation that they will not remember, or shouldn't have said. Strange as it may seem, they don't.

At times the patient may groan and toss with the contractions. Her husband has been told that she will not recall anything. This is the time for him to repeat this to himself over and over again. He has never seen his wife drugged. He has never seen her hair so disheveled, and the short hospital gown is hardly flattering. But these are small things compared with the life his wife is about to bring into the world. Tomorrow she will have her hair combed, her makeup in place, and will wear a pretty nightgown.

The third shot is usually given when the patient is eight centimeters dilated (four fingers breadth) and it will relieve all remembrance of pain. This is the time when the expectant grandmother says, "She's hurting but just doesn't know it". Pain is knowing.

Individual drugs cannot be discussed in a primer for the lay reader. Different doctors in different sections of the country use their individual chosen regimes. The names of the drugs or combination of drugs would not mean anything to you. **The fact that they prevent excessive pain is the important thing.** Many good drugs are available. Your doctor's choice has been guided by his training and experience.

REGIONAL ANAESTHESIA

These are basically called saddle block, caudal, epidural, para-vetebral block, et cetera. Incidentally, if the doctor tells the patient she will receive a saddle block she may reply, "Thank goodness I'm not going to get a spinal!" In fact, the two are the same, and every doctor knows that each patient has a relative or friend who had one of two complications from her spinal, either "she was paralized" or "her back hurts her even now". The first statement is ridiculous, and the second is universal in that ninety-nine percent of women have back pain from time to time. Most of the back pain is caused by BENDING OVER for dish towels, diapers, husband's socks, and the like. Whether you are pregnant or not, you should SQUAT to pick up even small items.

With regional anaesthesias, oral or hypodermic medications are given in early labor as if you were a candidate for the method previously described. This shows the overlapping of the four basic ways to alleviate pain which were listed on page 37. A regional routine is not started until the patient is four centimeters dilated, and reaching this stage in labor may be painful, hence the medication. With any regional you are alert or semi-alert at the birth of the baby.

Though you may not desire this type of anaesthesia, there are times when you must take it. If you have a more than mild heart condition, if you have a full stomach of recently ingested food, or if you have a very premature baby, you are a definite candidate for a regional block.

Likewise, if you have chosen this type of anaesthesia, you cannot have it under some conditions. If you have a large baby and a borderline pelvis, if you have a large breech (buttocks coming first) presentation, or if this is your second baby plus and you are dilating too fast, this anaesthesia is often not used. Your doctor will probably use the hypodermic type of medication. Trust your doctor's judgment.

Chapter 14

Natural Childbirth . . .

Natural childbirth is basically childbirth without the aid of drugs or anaesthesia. It's proponents stress physical and mental relaxation.

In order to achieve relaxation during natural childbirth, practice breathing deeply while lying on your back with knees slightly drawn up (flexed). Take deep breaths and exhale slowly with either a hissing or soft blowing sound. Your breathing should be slow, rhythmic, and relaxed. Have your arms extended and relaxed by your sides with the hands open and the palms up. Practice breathing like this for some fifteen minutes daily.

During the breathing exercises, think how relaxed you are. Your feet feel heavy, your whole body feels relaxed, and soon you **are relaxed.** If your mind wanders, think or concentrate on a ceiling light fixture. Practice and practice over nine months. You will be surprised at the degree of control you have over your body in attaining this restful and relaxed state. Incidentally, this exercise also helps cure insomnia. (It will alleviate the tossing and tension you have at night, when you become a human computer for real or imaginary troubles.)

Even if you are not planning to follow the whole natural childbirth routine, the exercise will reduce pain and its resulting mental anxiety. Whether you receive medical shots or a regional block, the relaxation will help you progress to the point where medication is required. There are many books on the subject. Check with your local book store.

Most instructions for natural childbirth do not cover dilation from two centimeters (about ½ inch) to complete, when the cervix is opened some five inches in diameter allowing the baby to pass from the uterus into the birth canal (vaginal vault). It is seldom explained that this is the most painful part of labor. The muscles of the womb push the presenting part of the baby against the opening to achieve dilatation. The process of dilating can take quite a few hours, especially with first babies. Some hypodermic medication can be used in the latter stages of natural childbirth. Do not hesitate to request it.

Doctors who argue against natural childbirth refer to it as covered-wagon obstetrics because medical science can now alleviate pain without harming you or your baby. When you hit your thumb with a hammer, it hurts. You can practice relaxation from trauma all your life but the pain is still there. Relaxation, and self hypnosis to the contrary, pain is a reality of life. It can be mentally intensified or diminished, but it is a fact.

It is false to claim that the specific choice of drugs administered by your doctor will harm you or the baby. Your baby's condition at birth, as well as shortly after delivery is scored by an Apgar rating which observes how quickly the baby breaths and cries. The baby's reflexes are tested, and pulse rate checked. A healthy pink condition is noted. The top score for an Apgar is 10, with two points given for each condition described above. Any Apgar over seven is satisfactory. In most hospitals the rating is scored by a trained nurse or anaesthesiologist. This is a time-honored and valid test for the physical condition of your baby at birth and shortly after. The Apgar ratings are no better for babies born with natural childbirth than for those delivered with the aid of properly chosen medications and regional anaesthesias. There are established drugs that an experienced doctor knows will not harm your baby.

Choose whatever method of birth you desire but never give it first place in importance. The new life is the exciting fact and there will never be another baby like yours. The hearts of men and women are proud, and they would like to make the **event** of childbirth more important than the miracle of the baby. Out in the field of obstetrics, it is the **product** that is precious and not the method of delivery.

Husbands can be helpful in the labor room; their presence is calming and comforting. Shortly before actual birth of the baby, you will be taken into the delivery room and some patients want their husbands present at this time too. They believe that the birthing of the baby can be a deep-seated emotional experience for them, and that it will bind them closer to each other and the baby. This recalls the "old days" when expectant fathers actually delivered the babies. If this emotional premise is valid, then the olden days must have been the golden age of marriage; however, history does not substantiate this concept. Do not expect your husband's witnessing the baby's birth to materially alter your relationship any more than his watching you have an appendix removed or a tooth extracted. The birth of a baby is an earthy experience of blood, urine and feces. If you feel that the cords of your marriage need strengthening, do it by means of professional marriage counselling. Seek help before the wall of love and communication between you is too strong to tear down.

A fainting husband in the delivery room detracts from the attention being given you and your baby. (Incidentally a rare doctor only desires to watch his wife give birth to a child.) The possibilities of a negative response on the husband's part does not warrant his being there so you will have a "conversation piece" with friends.

Chapter 15

Induction of labor . . .

Induction of labor involves starting labor pains by medical procedures in the hospital. Certain difficulties of pregnancy such as toxemia or an Rh complication (see next chapter) can cause your doctor to decide in favor of an induction. These are specifics and will be explained in detail by the doctor.

But the most frequent reason for induction is the patient's convenience. An elective (convenience) induction is done only when the baby is firmly fixed in the pelvis and the cervix has begun to dilate (the cervix is 'ripe'), which is determined by a pelvic examination at the doctor's office when you are near term.

If you go over due date, you are very impatient and tired of being pregnant. Friends call with the cheery words, "haven't you gone yet". Don't urge your doctor to bring the baby because you think it is due. (More pressure is put on doctors about this than any other facet of obstetrics.) He knows you are anxious. If the examination shows that conditions are favorable, he may offer an induction.

"When the apple is ripe, it will fall" is true. Hasty obstetrics to please you or your kin can lead to complications. Pay no attention when friends tell you of cases that never went into labor. This is false information. And remember a good doctor will not do anything that may harm you or your baby, even though you try to pressure him with words and tears.

Chapter 16

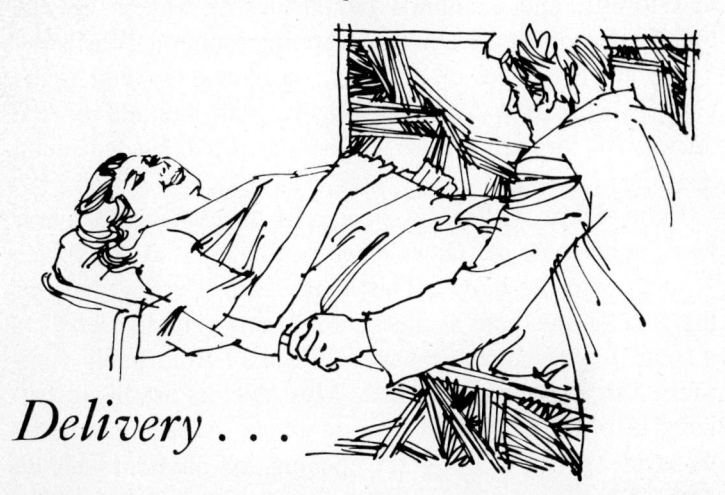

Delivery...

When the mouth of the womb is fully dilated (10 centimeters, five finger breadths, or called by your doctor completely dilated), the baby then is in the birthcanal (vagina). It must be stated that under the medical induced analgesia or in natural childbirth the patient will bear down as if she were going to have a bowel action. If a regional block is used, the patient has no sensation of this.

The abdominal muscles are used when bearing down. Under the medical analgesia she doesn't recall doing this;—it's not unlike a reflex action to your body. With natural childbirth you are instructed to take a deep breath, hold it, and bear down.

As the baby progresses through the birth canal it reaches the opening of the vagina, and there is a definite bulging of that area (called crowning). With first babies you are usually allowed to crown before you are taken to the delivery room. With second babies plus you are usually taken to the birth area a bit earlier to prevent your having the baby in the labor room (called a precipitious delivery).

You are cleansed by the nurse, drapped with sterile sheets and towels, and examined by the doctor who is dressed like the doctors you see in the operating room on Television. There are two types of birth; (a) spontaneous—that is the baby is expressed from the vagina with the aid of the doctor, (b) forceps—this instrument is a two bladed metal instrument.

Many years ago forceps were used only when the doctor was forced to do so. Older mothers still say that the doctor "had to take the baby". This is nonsense. Forceps fit over the side of the baby's cheek bones and actually serve as a splint to prevent the bones of the skull from being compressed in a spontaneous birth. Most doctors use his instrument in order to prevent brain damage. A baby pounding its head against the vaginal opening for an hour can do himself harm.

With first babies the patient wonders how the baby can "get out". In the past intercourse may have had some discomfort, so she thinks to herself how can anything as large as a baby's head pass through the birth canal.

The answer is best expressed by two points; (a) as you reach term the ovaries, tubes, and bladder have been pulled up by the growth of the foetus giving more room between the pelvic bones (b) as you approach term the blood vessels of the vagina increase allowing the vagina to expand.

With first babies the doctor usually makes an incision (an episiotomy). This is done for the following reasons; (a) a controlled incision heals better than a tear (b) it prevents the baby's head from being squeezed through a tight opening, and (c) it prevents tears in the muscles under the skin. Again, older females proudly say that they didn't have any stitches. They do not mention the fact that they feel as if everything were falling out every step they take.

Nor do they tell you that their gynecologist has told them that they have a relaxed vaginal outlet which must be repaired at a later date.

The stitches hurt. See the chapter on post partum care of them. They are not removed but dissolve.

Caesarean Section

A Caesarean section is performed by making an abdominal incision through the uterus to deliver the baby. In laymen terms, a Caesarean section is done for two reasons; Firstly, a normal vaginal delivery would endanger either your life or the baby's if your pelvis is too small for the baby to pass through. If you have a borderline (not very small but not up to average) pelvis the doctor may obtain an X-Ray of you and your baby in order to be certain that the pelvic measurements are adequate. He will tell you on the first examination what type of pelvis you have. Secondly, the placenta (afterbirth) can cause trouble by its location in the uterus. If it is down far ahead of the baby in the uterus, a Caesarean will have to be performed.

These are complications which your doctor will explain to you and your husband before the operation. In most cases Caesareans should not be done without consultation with another physician as both baby and mother have a more difficult time. If you have one section, all of your babies will probably have to be delivered this way. Usually you are offered a tubal ligation for sterilization purposes after your third section, but it isn't necessary in many cases. I have some patients who have had more than five sections. A Caesarean is more difficult than a normal vaginal delivery, but is not usually dangerous for you.

Chapter 17

The Rh factor and Rubella vaccination . . .

One of the topics most often discussed over the bridge table is the fact that one member of the group is Rh negative. Usual remarks by friends "who know" are (a) "You can have only two babies without getting into trouble", (b) "after the first baby one's chances of having a deformed baby are very great", and (c) "that's very bad".

The fact is that the Rh factor present in the blood of the mother is positive some eighty-five percent of the time. Since this is not a scientific dissertation, here are some simple facts.

1. If you are Rh negative and have never had a pregnancy or a blood transfusion with Rh positive blood, **forget it.**

2. If your husband is Rh negative and you are positive, **forget it.**

3. There is a shot that is given to mothers who are Rh negative with their first babies. If the baby is Rh Positive, the mother receives the injection within seventy-two hours after delivery and that assures her of not having an Rh complications with her next pregnancy.

4. If you are Rh negative and have had a baby before this shot was developed, blood samples will be taken several times during your pregnancy. These tests will determine whether or not your blood is building up an antibody titers. If it is, your doctor will discuss this with you and additional testing may be made on the amniotic fluid.

In "legal" abortions, it is important that the Rh factor be checked on the abortee. Many doctors have possibly failed to do so and some of these women with Rh negative blood will have trouble with a planned pregnancy.

RhoGam Rh-o(D) immune Globulin (humane) administered to the Rh negative woman within seventy-two hours after an Rh positive childbirth, miscarriage, or abortion prevents the blood disease in future pregnancies. It is in this way that the Rh problems with the babies can be eliminated within a single generation.

Your doctor has pamphlets about the Rh factor and will offer them to you. Write down any questions you have on the subject, and he will answer them honestly and to the point. Pregnant women often worry needlessly. Don't lose a night's sleep staring into darkness thinking of all the horrible things that are in store for your baby because you're Rh negative. Your husband is on his back snoring. Nudge him to turn over and go to sleep.

Rubella

The next most discussed complication to your baby is whether or not you have had the German measles (Rubella). In very early pregnancy it is a fact that if you have rubella your baby can have several defects.

Most women had rubella as children; but don't remember. Your doctor may take a blood sample on the first visit. If this is tested for that disease, your immunity or non-immunity will be determined. If you are pregnant, you should **not** receive the rubella vaccine. Harm may come to your baby even when the vaccine is received shortly before you become pregnant. Many doctors believe that a year should elapse between the vaccine and pregnancy. The present program of immunizing children will eliminate the problem of rubella in less than a generation.

Chapter 18

The hospital . . .

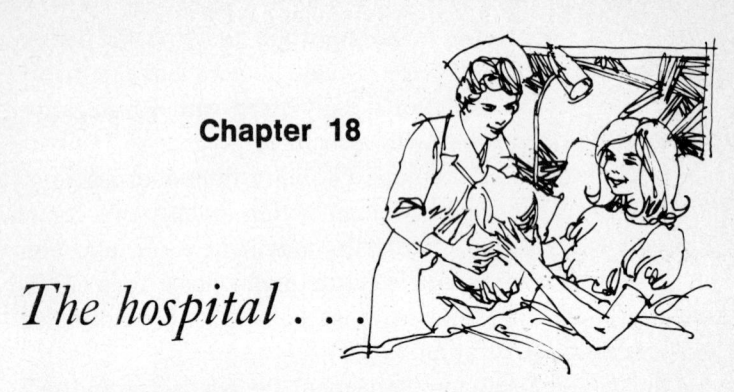

Information about hospitals may be helpful to you. Your doctor will often have a choice of one or two hospitals that he uses, and I strongly advise you not to argue with him about this. Friends will add pro and con gossip about every hospital. Your doctor knows which one will be best for you.

Patients frequently choose a hospital because of its newness, its appearance, or a favorite clerk. Unfortunately, the layman's choice often is based on which religious organization runs the hospital. For example, some Protestants ignorantly believe that a Catholic institution "lets the mother die and saves the baby". The only difference between a Catholic hospital and any other is that your doctor can not sterilize the patient simply because she does not want any more babies. Don't forget the hospital treatment is ordered by your doctor and not by the hospital staff. You must remember that **he** is responsible for you.

Your doctor judges the hospital by the medical facilities available in case an emergency arises. He is concerned with the type of help that is available if he needs an extra "pair of hands" in a difficult delivery. He is concerned with how fast the laboratory can type and cross-match blood and get it to the delivery room in an emergency. These emergencies do not occur often, but when they do they are vital for the well-being of you and your baby.

Preliminary Visit to the Hospital

When you are near term it is a good idea for you and your husband to visit the hospital. Time yourself so you will know how long the leisure drive will take. Find the admitting office. It is suggested that you and the father-to-be go to the maternity floor **during** normal visiting hours. You will learn the location of the obstetrical area and have the bonus of seeing the newborn babies through the glass window of the nursery. When you and your doctor have agreed on the hospital, you can go to the business office before the baby is due and make financial arrangements. Take your hospital policy or its number to the office. The personnel can tell you how much the policy will cover in an obstetrical case. This will allow you to "pay as you go" before birth of your baby. Most hospitals do not detain the patient in labor in the admitting office: they **do** ask the expectant father many questions about his wife's birthplace, religion, and so on. This is a necessity, but it can be handled many weeks before admittance. By checking with the hospital in advance, you will not have to cope with the institution's routine paper work machine at the time of admittance.

The end of nine months pregnancy is no surprise to the family. They have had many months to take care of the hospital bill, as well as their doctor's bill, before "D" day (delivery day). Obstetricians know the unpredictability of labor and delivery. They know that they are liable to be called away from everything from the office appointments to personal family crises. They do not complain. But they do desire the expectant parents to have made their financial arrangements before the baby is born.

Chapter 19

The expectant Grandmother . . .

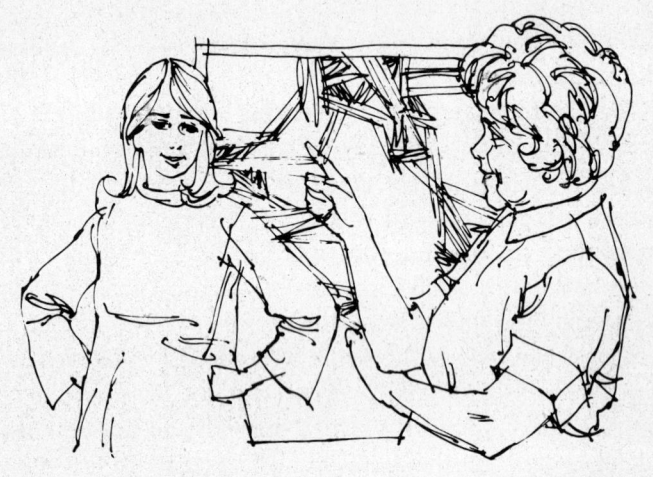

Bless grandmother. It will be a hard nine months for her, especially if this is her first grandchild. She is fortified with the wisdom learned from rearing a family. There is no substitute experience for this brand of learning. It is a hard and maturing school. Add love to wisdom and you have a dynamo of strength, prepared to help in every way. In the field of medicine, grandmother is smarter than she used to be, but not so smart as she should be. She is modern, but she is apt to remember all those old wives' tales. The more she thinks about them, the more real they seem. "Doctors don't know everything, you know. After all, has your doctor ever had a baby?"

Don't misunderstand me—I like mothers. I have one of my own. And I have learned to bounce right back after a serious run-in with a grandmother-to-be. They don't like obstetricians, they don't trust them, and they don't agree with them. This all adds up to lots of negative thinking. It can shake your faith in the whole world of medicine. After all, mother has had babies and your doctor has not. This fact can divide your loyalties between mother and doctor in no time.

Grandmother-to-be starts psychologically undermining you the moment she hears your news. She is happy, but "How do you feel? "Have you had much nausea?" she asks. The question has great impact because "mother was sick the whole nine months". Many, many women never experience nausea for reasons already explained (chapter 2), but this psychological suggestion from mother can trigger the pregnant one into real trouble. Mother's fears and anxieties are limitless. She has had many more friends who have had babies than you have. Their experiences pyramid into a vast storehouse of misinformation. You do not see your doctor very often, but you talk with mother frequently. Her prenatal propaganda can be treacherous.

It is time to be honest. We love mother, but your baby is your doctor's responsibility. You pay for the advice that he has been trained to give. He will not deceive you. He will stress the things that are important for your health as well as your baby's.

Ask mother to read this primer. She may not always agree, but she is smart, and we hope that she will see reason. Pregnancy is the same old nine months' affair, but the ways of coping have progressed. Don't let your mother cross up your line of communication with your doctor.

When delivery day arrives, grandmother-to-be is tense. She favors very heavy sedation. After the baby is delivered, everyone is happy. Grandmother too seems pleased and satisfied. But her calm moments are short. She cannot understand why her daughter is staying in the recovery room. She completely forgets that she was pushing for heavier sedation just an hour earlier.

The day that mother and baby leave the hospital is the day that the obstetrician and grandmother begin to agree. If you thought that grandmother knew all about helping your obstetrician, just wait until she starts helping the pediatrician. Unless, of course, she has learned the glorious lesson that occasionally she may be mistaken.

The truly wise grandmother can be a great help to you when you are home. Love and care come naturally to her. The baby needs her and so do you. Three generations make a rich and well-rounded family. A little planning and scheduling will coordinate family efforts and create a harmonious atmosphere for all. You and your baby need loving relatives and friends. There is depth of security for all in the big family circle.

Chapter 20

Postpartum hospital courses . . .

(Or "They Wake Me Up to Give Me a Sleeping Pill")

After the birth of the baby, your doctor will go to the fathers' waiting room. He will give the good news to your husband and family. It is advised TO CALL ONLY ONE OR TWO OTHER PERSONS when you go to the hospital. Most doctors advise husbands not to phone the family until the wife is taken to the delivery room. They will have adequate time to get there for the announcement and to see the newborn with you. If four people (plus or very seldom minus) accompany you to the hospital, the waiting room gets confused and crowded. Rather alarming advice vibrates around the area. Hospitals are for mother, baby, and father, and not a gathering of the clan. Visitors make frequent trips up and down the halls to the coffee machine or to the rest rooms. They can spread germs and interrupt an otherwise normally functioning hospital. Think of the patients who have had their babies. You will resent all the bustle when you are later admitted to your room to recuperate and you want rest and quiet.

Soon after the birth, a nurse will show your baby to his father through the glass window of the nursery. Father will get a good, long look at his fine, red-faced infant. The baby will have a pointed head and a flat forehead. Don't be dismayed. This is normal. In twenty-four hours he will be beautiful.

You will be taken to the recovery room. When you can drink water and are fairly alert you are taken to your own hospital room in the obstetrical area. Your family should not be alarmed that you spend 2-6 hours in the recovery room. All patients are kept in "recovery" until the vital signs like blood pressure and pulse rate are normal. This is not an expectation of complications; it is just good medicine. In your own room you will put on your pretty nightgown and be yourself again. Your doctor has written many many orders on your chart. These orders tell the nurses what to do for you from day to day, with special instructions for diet and other routines. Every obstetrician hears indignant words from patient and family about what "they" (the hospital staff) did or did not do last night. He knows what "they" did. He ordered it. All hospital food is bland, so don't expect to change this situation. Your doctor studies your chart before he talks with you. He knows all about your condition. If an unexpected complication develops, he is notified.

Your doctor will see you daily and he will answer the questions you have for him. **Write them down.** He will give you printed instructions as to your routine at home. Read these. Ask questions before the time for him to discharge you and the baby. The pediatrician will also see you daily, and you should ask him any questions that you may have about how to take care of your baby.

Friends think that you need many visitors while you are in the hospital. Visitors mean well, but in large numbers they are a plague to you, your family, and the hospital personnel. Some doctors routinely give patients a tranquilizer thirty minutes before visiting hours. The reason for this is obvious. Your stitches hurt, and the "baby blues" may be starting, but you must seem pleased to see them even though you are tired.

Baby blues is a condition often seen. About the third day the new mother feels the urge to cry. She is doing well, and her baby is normal, but she has a good crying jag. There is no cure for this. But it is helpful to understand that this is normal and that the mood will pass soon (see chapter 20)

With your first baby you will keep a very complete baby book. That's normal. With baby number two, you remember the date, the weight, and the sex. That's just as normal.

The new daddy needs a bit of advice about hospital gift shops: he shouldn't overbuy. These shops have the oldest cigars. How many of your friends smoke cigars anyway? There are other items which are expensive and nonessential. The father is happy, enthusiastic, and "what does the cost matter?" An "It's a Boy" sign on a small doll with a football and jersey is very tempting. It rarely gets home with you. If it does, you don't know what to do with it. Think before buying.

Chapter 21

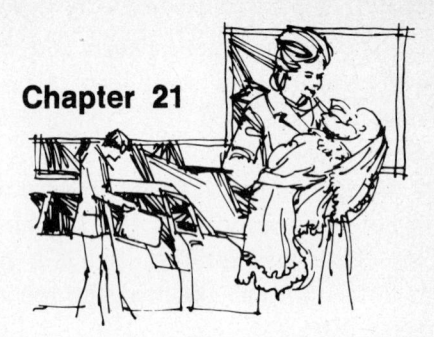

Going home

Your obstetrician usually gives you a complete pamphlet or sheet of do's and don't's after the birth of your baby. Read these carefully. When it is time to go home, he will have a talk with you. He wants you to ask him questions about his instructions. **Again,** write down your questions when you can take a break between baby's coming to your room and the many visitors. The latter should stay at home and write you notes, instead of spreading cheer and germs around your hospital room.

Incidentally, the visitors who arrange themselves around the multitude of flowers in your room will always ask you how you feel. Although you are tired and feel "let down" (baby blues), you have to act appreciative of their calling. If you just smile at your well-wishers and don't talk, you'll save energy and reduce a great deal of emotional tension. And please don't take all those flowers home. Have them sent to some room without flowers, or to the children's ward in the hospital. One of the hazards of loading up to depart, besides paying the bill, is that someone always turns over a vase containing cut flowers and water.

When driving home with your husband, be certain that he keeps his eyes on the road and not on the baby. After arriving home, everything is set for you except for one item: no visitors. Your husband can improvise two cardboard signs. One says Patient Resting. This is to go on your door from 10:00 A.M. to noon, and from 2:00 P.M. until 4:00. The other sign should be on the baby's nursery door. This sign **should** say Don't Breathe Over the Baby [germs again], Don't Touch, and Don't Make Noise. Actually all it can say is Baby Sleeping.

Your pediatrician will give you detailed instructions about handling the newborn. Follow them implicitly. If "problems" arise (they always do with the first-born) call his office and leave your number. He often makes his phone calls when he takes a break from office babies. Don't call your obstetrical doctor about the baby.

It can't be stressed too much that one small bundle of joy can beat four grandparents, mother, and father down to a state of exhaustion in a few days. If the offspring cries, everyone jumps. If the baby is quiet, one of you tiptoes into the room to see if he or she is breathing. In a changing world, babies remain eternally the same. They are miracles of wonder and tenderness. They are yours to mold and love. Parenthood is a great and marvelous work.

Stitches

The place where the doctor made the incision to enlarge the opening of the vagina is called an episiotomy. It can hurt. Pain pills ease the soreness, and a more-than-warm sitz bath in the tub is also very helpful. Fill the tub with four or five inches of water and sit in the same for twenty minutes three or four times a day. One may also use dry heat in conjunction with sitz baths. Make a cradle with a coat hanger so you don't burn the sheets and use a bedside lamp (60 watts) some eighteen inches from the area. Do this four or five times daily as long as you desire. WE AREN'T TRYING TO GIVE YOU A BURN OR A FLORIDA TAN, so don't have your husband purchase a special lamp or any infrared bulbs.

When you first awake in the morning, you will notice

that the incision is more painful than when you went to bed. This indicates that activity promotes healing as well as easing the pain. There is nothing better than proper exercise, but simply walking slowly around the bed or to the bathroom will help.

Some patients have a separation in the incision. This will heal in time. An episiotomy is not like an appendectomy incision, because it is never dry. There is the normal blood and some perspiration pouring over the area. One can't place a bandage dressing over the area, so healing is slower.

Fainting

You can prevent fainting or getting dizzy by following the same rules explained in chapter 10.

You Still Have a Tummy

It takes six weeks for the uterus to return to normal. Your doctor has told you when to start mild abdominal exercises. Too early exercises of the "stomach" will do no good in regaining abdominal tone. Girdles or abdominal supports should not be used unless prescribed by your doctor.

Care of the Breasts

Whether you breastfeed or not, some engorgement of the breasts is expected. A binder or a bra that is **specially fitted** by a clerk from a local surgical supply house should be used. A binder that prevents curvature of the breasts to the side will help. Check the position of the breasts by lying on your back. Place your right hand to the side of your **left** breast and vice versa. If there is a curve, the binder (or bra) is not adequate.

A binder may be improvised by holding your breast toward the breast bone (middle). Have someone use a diaper and pin this in place with large safety pins as you hold the breasts in this position. Engorgement can cause pain, chills and fever. Take aspirin if fever is present.

Bowels

If the baby is not breastfeeding ANY laxative is good. If you are eating normally, you should have an action every day. If you are breastfeeding ask your pediatrician about this, **before you leave the hospital.** A plain water enema may be taken at any time unless your doctor says otherwise.

Stairs

You may go up and down stairs. A change of environment is a great boost to your morale. Ask help if you feel faint. If you are dizzy, sit down at once.

Vaginal Bleeding

Vaginal bleeding will continue off and on for several weeks. If it stops and returns in a few days, don't be alarmed. Phone your doctor only if you are expelling blood clots THE SIZE OF AN ORANGE. The "night bleeding" often panics a patient, and she rushes to the hospital emergency room. This needless fright is often stimulated by some kin who say "you are hemorrhaging to death." Remember, it takes very little blood to cover a napkin or two.

Baby Blues

Usually while you are still at the hospital you feel as if everything has gone wrong. Your baby is healthy, you are in excellent condition, but you feel like crying. Your husband is five minutes late coming to the hospital, the nurse irritates you, and so does your doctor. Please have a good cry and get over this. There is no preventing these "baby blues" once they have started. A good cry is the only cure. Some think this temporary depression is due to the fact that the nine months of worrying are at an end. Everything is more or less all right, and you feel a let down. This condition is normal.

Early Ambulation

While in the hospital you will be encouraged to get out of bed as soon as possible. This prevents blood clots from forming in the pelvic blood vessels and lower limbs (thrombophlebitis). It also helps the womb to return to its normal size. It reduces the pain in your stitches, and keeps you from getting extremely weak.

Get up slowly to prevent fainting. Don't stay out of bed for a prolonged period of time, but get up often. Many older relatives will frown on this, but ignore them.

Diet

Follow any diet you wish unless your doctor makes exceptions. You should also drink plenty of fluids. This prevents bladder infections. It will also help with breastfeeding. Again, no female drinks an adequate supply of water. Eight glasses daily is strongly suggested.

BREAST FEEDING OR BOTTLE FEEDING?

You will receive much advice about the manner you should feed your baby. Both the breast feeding and the bottle feeding friends are as vigorous in their opinions as they are about their other instructions given you.

The following points may help you decide.

(1) "Breast feeding depends upon the size of your bosoms". This is not true. The full breasted female has more FAT tissue than her smaller bosomed friends. Basically the same amount of milk producing tissue is present in most females.

(2) "Breast-fed babies do better". In some cases this is true. Breast feeding does give the baby a few of the resistances against viral infections that the mother has built up in her blood stream.

(3) Breast feeding does aid the female organs in return-

ing to normalcy, but this isn't important enough to FORCE yourself to follow this schedule on the baby and to disregard necessary leisure time to get over the nine months. Your time with other children or your husband may be more important.

(4) Bottle feeding gives you time to relax and get out of the house later in your postpartum course. Breast feeding obviously hinders this at times.

(5) "You don't love your baby if you don't breast". This is ridiculous. This thought is continued by those who can breast feed without cracked nipples or other minor complications.

(6) "Breast feeding causes 'flat bosoms' when you are later dried up (lactation is suppressed)". This is said by the female who probably had breasts half way between the size of a golf ball placed on a fried egg. False!

So what do you do? Discuss this with your obstetrician while you are pregnant. Don't make a final decision until you have had your baby and discussed personal pros and cons with both your husband and your pediatrician. No baby doctor will force you to do so because with pressure applied, you will do a poor job. This is an individual decision and must be made by you and your particular circumstances.

Many obstetricians suggest you try nursing. Doctors can give medication to suppress lactation after you have gone home from the hospital just as easily and effective as they can during the hospital stay. There is no need to rush this decision.

Chapter 22

Old wives' tales and some random facts . . .

1. "This bleeding shows that the baby is deformed."

Not true. Why would a doctor try to stop the bleeding of early pregnancy if he suspected a malformed infant? One may have a spontaneous abortion (a miscarriage in the first three months of pregnancy) and expel the products of conception in spite of the bed rest, the hormone shots, and other measures taken, but this does not mean that the baby was deformed.

2. "Don't reach up with your arms, as it will cause the cord to be wrapped around the baby's neck."

Strange, but this is often said by very intelligent people. It's ridiculous. There is no connection between one's arms and the baby happily and securely floating around in the bag of waters.

3. "They say you can tell the sex of the baby by its heartbeat.

Impossible. The baby's heartbeat changes often during the day. Some obstetricians get so tired of this question that they laughingly say, "Sounds like a boy." If it is a male child, the parents spread the news that their doctor was able to diagnose the sex before birth: "My doctor told me, so I know it can be done." They missed the humor in the doctor's expression.

4. "You are carrying your baby low, so it's going to be a boy."

Not fact. Ninety-nine percent of your friends tell you that you are carrying the baby low. The force of gravity is down, and since that is where most of your prenatal pain is, you agree (see **pressure pains** described in chapter 7).

5. "He had to 'take' the baby with forceps."

Rarely do we **have** to use forceps. They are utilized on an optional basis to act as a splint for the foetus' skull. They fit over the cheek-bones of the unborn infant and prevent undue squeezing of the head as it passes through the vaginal vault. If you have premature baby, the doctor usually uses forceps to protect the premature skullbones from pressing too hard against the brain of the three-pound-plus-or-minus infant.

6. "You look so frail, you'll have a hard time."

This is usually said by some fat person who wishes she didn't have an eating problem. Fat is one of the complications of delivery (see chapter 8 on diet).

7. "Your baby will come when the moon is full."

This is false. The doctor wishes it were true so that he could plan his night schedule accordingly.

8. "The doctor had to 'bring on labor' when I had my baby! I would never have started."

See chapter 15, "Induction of Labor." The doctor probably did an induction because this patient called him many times in false labor.

9. "If you don't walk a mile a day you will have a hard time."

See pressure pains in chapter 7.

10. "You must eat for two" or "Just this one time won't hurt you."

When you are starving with the abnormal desire for food that pregnancy brings, this is like offering a drink to the alcoholic who is trying to stop his habit. Your willpower is strained. The temptation put before you can harm both you and the baby (see chapter 8 on diet).

11. "Eat Liver. It builds you up."

Many years ago patients with pernicious anemia had to eat liver in order to stay alive. It had to be consumed raw as cooking removed the beneficial elements. The rumor persists that "liver is good for you." In fact it harms you, because it is greasy, it has a high cholesterol content, and it contains neculo-proteins which are detrimental.

Chapter 23

Miscellaneous tips . . .

Smoking
If you smoke, DON'T STOP while you are pregnant. Your appetite will increase and you will be more prone to gain weight.

Alcohol
A social drink does you no harm if it doesn't break down your willpower to resist food. Taking an occasional drink if you are in the habit of doing so is all right. But remember the caloric content is high.

Douching
The variation of doctors' opinions about douching is very great. A gentle, plain water douche with a very clean (semi-sterilized) soft nozzle is often allowed once a week, from the fourteenth week of pregnancy through the thirtieth week.

Intercourse
Not more than once every week, and then not when your period would be due if you weren't pregnant. No intercourse from the sixth month to term.

Beauty Parlor
Go. It will lift your spirits. But don't listen to the chatter about pregnancy while there. Beauty parlors are "cells"

to undermine obstetricians. I think this is where "they" (as in "they say") work and are patrons.

Trips

Good for you if you don't take the holiday as an excuse to overdo or overeat. No trips after the 28th week.

Sunbathing

A good tan will lift your spirits.

Tub Bathing

Relaxing. As you grow larger, use caution getting in and out of the tub. Stop tub baths at the thirty-fourth week of pregnancy, use the shower after that.

Dentist

Any necessary dental work can be done. An infected tooth can cause complications.

X-Rays

Ask your doctor.

Medications

In the U. S. A. there are very few medicines sold that will harm your baby. But always ask your obstetrician on one of the routine trips before taking nonprescribed medicine.

Driving Your Car

Drive until you feel awkward and then stop.

Moving

Control your nesting instinct and go to mother's or a friend's house. Your husband will surprise you in his choice of what goes where in the new house or apartment. It is very important that you should not help with the moving.

Shopping

No prolonged trips. Shop when it is cool. Take your husband along; he'll see that it's a brief outing.

SHOPPING FOR THE BABY

The following list includes basic items which should be bought for your baby. Climate and season determine the exact kind. This is a plus or minus list:

4-6 receiving blankets
2-4 Kimonoes
4-6 nightgowns
4-6 rubber pants
2-3 dozen diapers (if you use diaper service)
4 safety pins
3-4 nightgowns
4-6 undershirts
6 crib sheets
1-2 crib blankets
1 box of waterproof pads
1 set of crib bumper pads
3-4 bathtowels
3-4 washcloths
4 teething bibs
8-10 eight-ounce bottles
2-4 four-ounce bottles
1 bottle brush
Sterilizer kit (electric preferred)
Bottle warmer
Alcohol
Q-tips
Cotton balls
Small gauze pads
Baby lotion or oil
Baby soap
Diaper bag
Soiled clothes bag

Chapter 24

Birth control...

After the birth of the baby it is not advisable to have intercourse until the baby is six weeks of age and you have had your postpartum check with your doctor. Birth control will be one of the main subjects you will wish to discuss with him. There are probably more old wives' tales about the methods of birth control than there are about delivery.

The Pill

The pill has taken much abuse. Cancer, weight gain, blood clots, falling hair, and an early menopause have been blamed on the pill. Many of these conditions have made magazine and newspaper headlines. Rumors have buzzed from hairdryer to hairdryer in the beauty salon and from bridge table to bridge table in the home, gathering speed wherever the girls meet.

The following statements about the pill are definite and, in my belief, are the opinions of the majority of obstetricians and gynecologists:

1. The pill is safe.

2. The pill is effective if taken as directed. It prevents ovulation, so conception is impossible if pills are taken regularly. After the birth of the baby, patients are told to start the pill five days **after** their first normal period begins. This menstruation period will be about six to ten weeks

after delivery. Take the pill daily. After the first prescription of twenty-one pills (twenty-eight with some brands) is taken, DON'T GO OVER A WEEK WITHOUT RESTARTING YOUR NEXT CYCLE OF PILLS. Start again on schedule irrespective of the presence or absence of vaginal bleeding.

When you forget to take the pill, or drop it in the commode, take two the following night and don't worry. It may be practical for you to tape your pill container to the toothpaste tube. When you brush your teeth at bedtime, you will automatically remember the pill. If you have forgotten the pill for two or more days, wait until you have a **normal** period and restart according to your beginning instructions. Of course, you can become pregnant during this lapsed time.

3. The person who says the pill is making her fat usually makes this statement while munching on a piece of chocolate pie. It is a crutch for the fat person. This is akin to the "everything I eat turns to fat" statement. It is true that one may experience temporary fluid retention and mild tension while taking this medication. If this condition exists, the doctor will prescribe "fluid pills" (diuretics) which will relieve the symptoms.

4. Some patients complain that the pill makes them nervous. In the absence of fluid retention, consider whether or not you are normally tense. Is your husband causing problems? Are the bills piling up? Are the normal products of conception running around the house trying to break the sound barrier?

5. "Break-through" bleeding may occur. This is vaginal bleeding which may occur while you are taking the pill as scheduled. It is not dangerous and may be controlled

by taking two pills instead of one for the rest of the twenty-one (or twenty-eight) days. Your doctor may wish to change your brand before you start the next month's supply. This unscheduled bleeding is a big problem to your doctor because you call him, call him, and call him. To repeat a statement used before, blood is red and vaginal bleeding makes most females push the emergency button. Don't. Follow the instructions above.

6. Nausea occurs in some patients during the first month of the medication. If this continues the second month a change of brand may be advised.

7. It is true that all patients cannot take this medication. A three month trial period may prove that you are an exception to the usual patient in which case another method will be prescribed.

8. Most mothers are very dubious about the pill. It wasn't present in their childbearing years. They are vehicles for many untrue tales about the harm the pill will do their daughters. I'm not certain that some big industries don't abate this rumor as the birth rate of this country is falling, and possibly the big companies (some) were geared for a population explosion. Most doctors have their wives and/or daughters on the pill to control their families.

The I.U.D. (intrauterine device)
An I.U.D. is a plastic device (coil, crab, look et cetera) inserted by the doctor into your cervix. The I.U.D. is put in place DURING your period. There are several objections to this. Some four percent (plus or minus different statistics) become pregnant inspite of the I.U.D. The same number experience abdominal cramping and bleeding.

The Foams and Jellies
Spermicidal foams and jellies are available in all drug

stores. They work by killing the sperm in the vagina and are about sixty-five percent effective. Many patients declare this method is effective until they try to get pregnant and find there was a sterility problem present all the time.

The Diaphragm

The diaphragm is about ninety-five percent efficient and before the advent of the pill, was the most widely used method. The diaphragm is fitted for the vaginal canal by the doctor and explained to you by his nurse. It is used with a spermicidal jelly and must be inserted before intercourse and allowed to remain in the vagina at least six hours after an exposure.

Condoms

Rubbers vary in their effectiveness due to two factors; (a) whether they break or not. (b) if the male partner will extract his organ from the vagina shortly after reaching a climax before the penis shrinks in size allowing some of the sperm to escape from the top of the rubber.

Tubal Ligation

Tubal ligation is an operation for sterilization that involves opening the abdominal cavity and tying off the two tubes which carry the egg from the ovary for fertilization, thus making conception impossible. It is a major operation as all operations are when the abdominal cavity is opened. If you don't have diabetes, heart trouble or some other serious illness, ask your husband to have a vasectomy.

Vasectomy

Vasectomy is a method of male sterilization in which the vas deferens in the scrotal sac is tied so that no sperm are present in the semen. A minute incision is made under local anaesthesia and the postoperative pain is practically nil. The procedure is minor surgery. The cost is minimal in comparison to that of a tubal ligation. Husbands shy away from this because they have heard that it will harm their manhood. Nonsense. This is another old wives tale (old husband's tale—?) which goes from barber chair to barber chair and from poker table to poker table. Why should a wife go through a MAJOR operation for birth control when the husband can easily go to his doctor's office on Saturday, have his vasectomy, and return to work after this MINOR procedure on Monday?